Controlling Your Blood Sugar Level

Leonard Dalton

Contents

Introduction

"Controlling Your Blood Sugar Level" is intended to be your ultimate reference for understanding and properly controlling your blood sugar levels. Whether you have diabetes, prediabetes, or just wish to live a healthy lifestyle, the information on these pages will empower you to take charge of your health.

In today's fast-paced world, when processed meals and sedentary lives are the norm, it is critical to prioritize our health, especially when it comes to blood sugar control. Elevated blood sugar levels may result in a variety of health concerns, including diabetes, heart disease, and renal difficulties. However, by implementing the appropriate tactics and making smart food choices, you may drastically lower your risk and live a more happy life.

Throughout this book, we will look at the science behind blood sugar regulation, the effect of various meals on blood sugar levels, and practical recommendations for staying within a safe range. You will receive vital information that will help you make well-informed choices about your nutrition and lifestyle, from understanding the significance of carbs, proteins, and fats to studying the advantages of regular physical exercise.

We will discuss the numerous obstacles that people experience when it comes to controlling their blood sugar levels. With so much contradicting information and fad diets available today, it's critical to differentiate reality from fiction. We will refute common myths and provide you with evidence-based solutions for regulating blood sugar levels that have been shown to be beneficial.

This book will also give you with useful tools and information to help you on your way to better health. You'll discover meal planning, recipe ideas, and portion management advice to help you enjoy tasty and healthy meals while keeping your blood sugar levels under control. We will also discuss the significance of monitoring and recording your blood sugar levels, which will enable you to make changes and assess the effect of your decisions on your general health.

Remember that regulating your blood sugar level is more than merely following tight diets or using short-term remedies. It's a way of life shift that emphasizes your long-term health and well-being. By using the ideas discussed in this book, you will not only be able to control your blood sugar levels, but you will also improve your general vigor and quality of life.

Join me on this revolutionary path to optimum health and discover how to confidently negotiate the complexity of blood sugar regulation. Let us go on a journey that will lead to better health, more energy, and a brighter future.

Chapter 1

Understanding Blood Sugar and Its Effects on Health

Introduction:

In this first chapter, we will build the groundwork for your road to properly regulating your blood sugar levels and maintaining your health. Understanding the fundamentals of blood sugar, its importance, and the variables that control it is critical for making educated food and lifestyle decisions. So, let's take a look at the interesting world of blood sugar and how it affects your general health.

1.1 Blood Sugar Research:

To appreciate the significance of blood sugar regulation, we must first grasp what blood sugar, or glucose, is and how it works in our bodies. Glucose is a form of sugar that acts as our cells' principal source of energy. It is derived from the meals we eat, particularly carbs, and is carried via the bloodstream to be used by numerous organs and tissues.

1.2 Insulin's Function:

Insulin is critical in controlling blood sugar levels. Insulin, which is produced by the pancreas, functions as a key that unlocks the cells, enabling glucose to enter and be utilized as fuel. Insulin also aids in the storage of extra glucose in the liver for later usage when blood sugar levels fall. However, in disorders such as diabetes, the body's capacity to create or use insulin properly is hindered, resulting in high blood sugar levels.

1.3 Imbalanced Blood Sugar Levels' Consequences:

When our blood sugar levels stay continuously high, it might have a negative impact on our health. Chronic high blood sugar, which is often linked with illnesses such as type 2 diabetes, may cause long-term damage to blood vessels, neurons, and organs. This raises the chances of developing heart disease, stroke, renal difficulties, eyesight loss, and other consequences. Hypoglycemia, or very low blood sugar levels, may induce dizziness, disorientation, and even loss of consciousness.

1.4 Blood Sugar Control Is Critical:

It is critical to maintain healthy blood sugar levels for general health and well-being. Whether you have diabetes, prediabetes, or wish to avoid developing these problems, maintaining good blood sugar management may help you live a happier, more enjoyable life. Blood sugar balance contributes to increased energy, better weight control, greater mental clarity, and a lower chance of long-term issues.

1.5 Blood Sugar Level Influencing Factors:

Blood sugar levels may be influenced by a variety of variables, including food choices, physical activity, stress levels, medicines, and general lifestyle. Understanding these elements and their influence on blood sugar management will enable you to make educated choices and take the required actions to keep blood sugar levels steady.

1.6 Blood Sugar Levels and Target Ranges:

Regular blood sugar testing is required to evaluate your progress and make any modifications. We will go through the various ways of blood sugar monitoring, such as at-home self-monitoring and laboratory testing, as well as the goal ranges to strive for in certain scenarios.

Conclusion:

You have taken an important step in controlling your blood sugar levels by understanding the foundations of blood sugar and its effect on health. In the following chapters, we will look at food options, physical activity guidelines, and other lifestyle changes that may help you attain and keep your blood sugar under control. Remember that information is power, and by knowing the science underlying blood sugar management, you will be better positioned to make health-enhancing decisions. So, let's continue this fascinating adventure together and discover the keys of good blood sugar management.

Chapter 2

Diet's Role in Blood Sugar Control

Introduction:

In Chapter 2, we'll look at how diet may help you regulate your blood sugar levels. Making educated and attentive eating choices may have a significant influence on our blood sugar management and general health. You will be able to construct a well-balanced eating plan that promotes optimum blood sugar management if you understand how various foods impact blood sugar and learn practical dietary methods.

2.1 Carbohydrate Influence:

Carbohydrates are the key macronutrient that has a large impact on blood sugar levels. Carbohydrates are broken down into glucose, which enters the circulation and boosts blood sugar levels. However, not all carbs are the same. We'll look at the glycemic index (GI) and glycemic load (GL) concepts to better understand how various carbs are digested and absorbed, and how they affect blood sugar levels differently.

2.2 Selecting the Correct Carbohydrates:

It is important to pick carbs intelligently in order to maintain stable blood sugar levels. We'll talk about how important it is to choose complex carbs that are high in fiber, such as whole grains, legumes, fruits, and vegetables. Because of their delayed digestion and absorption, these carbs have a smaller influence on blood sugar, delivering prolonged energy and facilitating better glycemic control.

2.3 Carbohydrate, Protein, and Fat Balance:

Combining carbs with appropriate protein and healthy fats may help decrease glucose absorption, reducing blood sugar increases. We will look at the advantages of include lean proteins like chicken, fish, and tofu in your diet, as well as healthy fats like nuts, seeds, avocados, and olive oil.

2.4 Meal Planning and Portion Control:

Maintaining portion control is critical for efficiently regulating blood sugar levels. We will present practical portion management suggestions and methods, such as utilizing smaller dishes, measuring portions, and being careful of portion sizes while eating out. We will also go over the necessity of meal planning and preparing well-balanced meals with a range of nutrients to maintain stable blood sugar levels throughout the day.

2.5 Fiber's Function:

Dietary fiber is well-known for its many health advantages, including its ability to improve blood sugar regulation. We will investigate the impact of soluble and insoluble fiber on digestion and blood sugar management. You will learn about high-fiber foods and how to include them into your meals to improve glycemic management.

2.6 Hydration and Blood Sugar Control:

Staying hydrated is important for general health, including blood sugar management. We'll talk about how important water is and how it affects blood sugar levels. We will also discuss the impact of sugary drinks and alcohol on blood sugar levels, as well as practical suggestions for choosing better beverage choices.

Conclusion:

You learned a lot about the function of nutrition in blood sugar management in Chapter 2. You can make educated dietary decisions if you understand how various nutrients, particularly carbs, protein, and fats, affect blood sugar levels. Balanced carbs, fiber-rich meals, portion management, and keeping hydrated are all important components of a well-rounded dietary plan that promotes stable blood sugar levels. The importance of regular physical exercise and its good effects on blood sugar regulation will be discussed in the next chapter. So, let us continue on this path to optimum health, where diet and lifestyle come together to produce a balanced and satisfying existence.

Chapter 3
The Benefits of Physical Activity in Blood Sugar Control

Introduction:

In Chapter 3, we'll look at the clear benefits of physical exercise for blood sugar control. Regular exercise and physical activity are not only useful for keeping a healthy weight and promoting cardiovascular health, but they also play an important role in managing blood sugar levels. This chapter will help you understand how various forms of physical activity affect blood sugar management and provide you with practical techniques for incorporating exercise into your daily routine.

3.1 Exercise's Benefits for Blood Sugar Control:

Exercise has a significant influence on blood sugar control. Physical exercise boosts insulin sensitivity, enabling cells to use glucose more efficiently. It also encourages weight reduction, which improves blood sugar management and lowers the chance of developing type 2 diabetes. Furthermore, exercise helps to improve cardiovascular health, mental well-being, and general energy levels.

3.2 Exercise Types and Their Effects on Blood Sugar:

Blood sugar levels are affected differently by different forms of exercise. Aerobic workouts, such as brisk walking, running, cycling, and swimming, aid in blood sugar control by raising insulin sensitivity and stimulating glucose absorption by muscles. Resistance training, such as weightlifting and bodyweight exercises, may help regulate blood sugar levels by increasing lean muscle mass, which assists in glucose metabolism. We will look at the advantages of aerobic and strength workouts, as well as how to integrate a well-rounded fitness plan into your daily routine.

3.3 Exercise Timing and Duration:

Exercise timing and duration might also have an effect on blood sugar levels. Exercise before and after meals may help manage blood sugar rises by increasing glucose absorption and utilization. We will advise you on when to exercise in relation to meals for optimal benefit. We will also go through the suggested length and frequency of exercise for maintaining consistent blood sugar management.

3.4 Strategies for Overcoming Exercise Barriers:

Overcoming barriers and sticking to a regular fitness program might be difficult at times. We will discuss typical hurdles to exercising, such as a lack of time, motivation, or physical restrictions, and provide practical solutions to these issues. You will learn how to create realistic objectives, locate enjoyable activities, and integrate physical exercise into your everyday life in a manner that works for you.

3.5 Blood Sugar Control During Exercise:

It is critical to keep your blood sugar levels steady throughout exercise for your safety and performance. We will go over the necessity of checking blood sugar levels before, during, and after exercise, as well as tactics for avoiding hypoglycemia (low blood sugar) and hyperglycemia (high blood sugar) when exercising. This involves changing medication doses, eating healthy snacks, and keeping hydrated.

3.6 Creating a Balanced Lifestyle: Nutritional and Physical Activity Synergy:

Chapter 3 finishes by highlighting the relevance of diet and exercise synergy in blood sugar regulation. You will improve your blood sugar management and general well-being by combining a balanced food plan from Chapter 2 with a regular exercise regimen. We'll talk about how diet and exercise work together to keep blood sugar levels constant, and we'll give you some practical strategies for incorporating both into your daily routine.

Conclusion:

The unquestionable power of physical exercise in blood sugar regulation was underlined in Chapter 3. Regular exercise has a variety of advantages, including better insulin sensitivity, weight control, cardiovascular health, and general well-being. You may leverage the favorable benefits of physical activity on blood sugar management by adding aerobic and resistance workouts into your regimen, scheduling exercise effectively, and overcoming hurdles. The relevance of stress management and sleep in maintaining stable blood sugar levels will be discussed in the next chapter. So, let us continue on this revolutionary path to optimum health, where lifestyle elements interact to produce a balanced and full existence.

Chapter 4

Stress Management and Sleep for Blood Sugar Stability

Introduction:

In Chapter 4, we'll look at the often-overlooked but critical role of stress management and sleep in maintaining stable blood sugar levels. Chronic stress and insufficient sleep may have a major influence on blood sugar control, making it critical to recognize their consequences and develop appropriate management techniques. You may improve your overall blood sugar management and well-being by reducing stress and emphasizing regular sleep.

4.1 Stress's Influence on Blood Sugar Levels:

Stress, whether physical, mental, or psychological, causes the body to respond with a series of hormonal reactions that might affect blood sugar levels. Stress chemicals such as cortisol and adrenaline may cause blood sugar levels to rise as the body prepares for a "fight or flight" reaction. Stress, whether short-term or long-term, may disturb blood sugar homeostasis and lead to insulin resistance. We will investigate the relationship between stress and blood sugar dysregulation and provide stress management solutions.

4.2 Stress Management Methods:

Maintaining normal blood sugar levels requires the use of stress management strategies. We'll talk about mindfulness meditation, deep breathing techniques, yoga, and participating in hobbies or activities that promote relaxation. You may reduce the detrimental effect of stress on blood sugar management by adding stress reduction practices into your everyday routine.

4.3 Sleep and Blood Sugar Control:

Sleep deprivation may disturb the body's hormonal balance and have a detrimental impact on blood sugar management. Sleep deprivation has been linked to increased insulin resistance, elevated blood sugar levels, and an increased chance of developing diabetes. We will discuss the significance of putting restful sleep first, as well as suggestions for improving sleep hygiene and developing a good sleep pattern.

4.4 Sleeping Suggestions:

We will go through practical advice and tactics for improving sleep quality. This involves creating a sleep-friendly atmosphere, sticking to a regular sleep schedule, reducing electronic device exposure before bed, and practicing relaxing methods. You may increase the length and quality of your sleep by adding these practices into your evening routine, which will have a good influence on blood sugar management.

4.5 Mind-Body Blood Sugar Management Techniques:

Biofeedback, progressive muscle relaxation, and guided visualization are examples of mind-body therapies that may help with blood sugar control. These techniques aid in stress reduction, relaxation, and general well-being. We will discuss the advantages of adding mind-body practices into your everyday routine as well as how to do so successfully.

4.6 A Holistic Approach to Blood Sugar Management:

Chapter 4 continues by emphasizing the significance of taking a comprehensive strategy to blood sugar management that includes variables other than food and exercise. You are adopting a complete approach to boosting your blood sugar control and general health by including stress management and emphasizing restful sleep. The interconnection of these lifestyle variables and their cumulative influence on blood sugar stability will be emphasized.

Conclusion:

We discussed the importance of stress management and sleep in maintaining stable blood sugar levels in Chapter 4. Chronic stress and sleep deprivation may affect blood sugar homeostasis and lead to insulin resistance. You may improve your well-being even more by employing stress-reduction tactics, emphasizing healthy sleep, and taking a holistic approach to blood sugar management. The need of frequent monitoring and medication management for diabetics will be discussed in the next chapter. So, let us continue on this illuminating path toward optimum health, where lifestyle variables and medical treatments combine to produce a balanced and joyful existence.

Chapter 5

Medication Management and Blood Sugar Monitoring

Introduction:

In Chapter 5, we will discuss the significance of frequent blood sugar monitoring and medication management for diabetics. Monitoring blood sugar levels and managing medications properly are critical components of obtaining and maintaining good blood sugar management. You may take an active part in maintaining your blood sugar levels and general health by learning the many monitoring techniques, goal ranges, and prescription alternatives available.

Methods for Monitoring Blood Sugar:

Regular blood sugar monitoring gives essential information about your body's reaction to food, activity, medication, and other variables. We will go through several blood sugar monitoring techniques, such as glucometer self-monitoring at home, continuous glucose monitoring (CGM) devices, and laboratory testing. You will learn about the advantages, disadvantages, and proper frequency of each technique, allowing you to make educated judgments on the best monitoring strategy for your circumstances.

5.2 Blood Sugar Target Ranges:

It is critical to understand target blood sugar levels in order to maintain optimum blood sugar management. The suggested goal ranges for fasting blood sugar, pre-meal blood sugar, post-meal blood sugar, and HbA1c values will be discussed. You will obtain a thorough grasp of the desirable blood sugar objectives, as well as how they help to lowering the risk of problems and attaining long-term health.

5.3 Medication Administration:

Medication is very important in controlling blood sugar levels in diabetics. We will go through the many forms of diabetic drugs, such as oral pills and insulin, as well as their mechanisms of action and the need of adhering to recommended regimens. You will learn about the possible adverse effects of medications, when to take them, and how to incorporate medication management into your daily routine.

5.4 Lifestyle Changes and Medication:

Lifestyle changes such as nutrition, exercise, stress management, and sleep work in tandem with medication to improve blood sugar control. We will look at how lifestyle variables might affect drug efficacy and the necessity of communicating openly with healthcare experts about lifestyle changes. Understanding the synergistic link between lifestyle changes and medication management can enable you to make more educated choices and achieve improved blood glucose control.

Management of Hypoglycemia and Hyperglycemia:

Hypoglycemia (low blood sugar) and hyperglycemia (high blood sugar) are both possible dangers for diabetics. We will go through the indications, symptoms, and treatment options for various illnesses. You will learn how to diagnose and manage hypoglycemia using glucose sources such as pills or snacks, as well as when to seek medical attention. Similarly, we will discuss hyperglycemia management techniques, such as medication adjustments, dietary changes, and lifestyle changes.

5.6 Working with Medical Professionals:

Collaboration with healthcare experts such as physicians, nurses, dietitians, and diabetes educators is required for accurate blood sugar monitoring and medication management. We will talk about the necessity of getting frequent check-ups, discussing honestly about blood sugar trends, making medication modifications, and seeking professional help when necessary. You may improve your blood sugar management and general well-being by actively engaging in your healthcare team.

Conclusion:

The importance of blood sugar monitoring and medication management for diabetics was stressed in Chapter 5. You may take charge of your blood sugar management and lower the risk of problems by frequently checking blood sugar levels, knowing goal ranges, and properly managing medication. Collaboration with healthcare providers and adopting required lifestyle changes improves the efficacy of drug management. The significance of support networks and self-care in sustaining long-term blood sugar management will be discussed in the next chapter. So, let us continue on this empowering path to optimum health, where information, cooperation, and self-empowerment come together to build a balanced and full existence.

Chapter 6

Long-Term Blood Sugar Control Support Systems and Self-Care

Introduction:

In Chapter 6, we'll look at how support networks and self-care may help you maintain long-term blood sugar management. Living with diabetes may be difficult, but with the correct support and self-care techniques, you can make the road easier. You may maintain optimum blood sugar management and live a satisfying life with diabetes by developing a strong support network, using self-care practices, and prioritizing your well-being.

6.1 The Value of Support Systems:

Individuals with diabetes benefit greatly from having a support system in place. We will talk about the many types of support available, such as family, friends, healthcare professionals, and diabetic support groups. You will learn how to articulate your requirements, request help when needed, and take use of the emotional, educational, and practical support available from your network.

6.2 Establishing a Support System:

Building a support network entails actively seeking out people who can provide understanding, encouragement, and direction. We will look at ways to strengthen your support network, such as visiting diabetic support groups, interacting with online forums, and having open talks with loved ones. You may improve your mental well-being and diabetes control by surrounding yourself with people who understand your path.

6.3 Self-Care Techniques:

Self-care is critical in treating diabetes and keeping blood sugar levels under control. We'll talk about several self-care methods that enhance physical, emotional, and mental well-being. Adopting a balanced diet, participating in regular physical exercise, successfully managing stress, prioritizing sleep, and adding relaxation methods into your routine are all part of this. You will discover how self-care activities may improve blood sugar management and general quality of life.

Diabetes and Emotional Well-Being:

Blood sugar regulation is intimately related to emotional well-being. We will look at the emotional elements of diabetes, such as the effects of stress, anxiety, depression, and diabetes-related suffering. You will learn coping skills for these emotions, as well as how to seek professional assistance when required and incorporate stress management approaches into your everyday life. Improving your mental well-being can help you regulate your blood sugar levels more successfully.

6.5 Diabetes and Lifestyle Changes:

Living with diabetes often necessitates lifestyle changes. We will discuss common difficulties and provide solutions to them. This involves controlling diabetes when traveling, negotiating social settings, and adjusting to changes in habits or locations. You can successfully tackle these lifestyle changes while maintaining excellent blood sugar control if you arm yourself with the proper tools and information.

6.6 Recognizing Success and Remaining Motivated:

Recognizing your accomplishments and keeping motivated are critical for long-term blood sugar management. We'll talk about how important it is to celebrate minor accomplishments and create realistic objectives. You will learn how to remain motivated, measure your progress, and include positive reinforcement into your journey. You may keep a positive outlook and remain dedicated to your blood sugar control by recognizing and applauding your victories.

Conclusion:

The need of support networks and self-care in sustaining long-term blood sugar management was underlined in Chapter 6. Building a solid support network, practicing self-care, and prioritizing emotional well-being are all critical components of successful diabetes control. You may handle the obstacles of diabetes with confidence and maintain optimum blood sugar control by seeking help, practicing self-care practices, and celebrating your accomplishments. In the last chapter, we will reflect on your transforming journey and provide some concluding insights on living a healthy and satisfying life with diabetes. So join me on this powerful path to optimum health, where support, self-care, and resilience combine to create a life of well-being and enjoyment.

Chapter 7

Reflections on a Balanced and Fulfilling Diabetes Life

Introduction:

We'll take a time in Chapter 7 to reflect on the remarkable journey you've made in regulating your blood sugar levels and living a balanced and fulfilled life with diabetes. Throughout this book, we've looked at food, exercise, stress management, medication management, support networks, and self-care practices as they relate to blood sugar control. It is now time to pull everything together and reflect on the lessons gained, the progress accomplished, and the road ahead to ongoing success.

7.1 Accepting the Journey:

Diabetes is a lifetime adventure that needs constant learning and adaptability. We'll talk about the obstacles you've encountered, the tenacity you've shown, and the personal development you've experienced along the road. You may build a positive mentality that will move you ahead by enjoying the trip and seeing it as a chance for progress and self-discovery.

7.2 Mindfulness and Gratitude:

Practicing gratitude and mindfulness may improve your general well-being significantly. We'll talk about how to cultivate appreciation for the benefits in your life, as well as how to use mindfulness practices to remain present and grounded. By adopting these techniques into your daily routine, you will be able to find pleasure in the little things and handle the ups and downs of living with diabetes with grace and perseverance.

7.3 Goal Setting and Revision:

Goal-setting is an important aspect of sustaining blood sugar management and personal development. We will look at how to develop SMART (Specific, Measurable, Achievable, Relevant, and Time-bound) objectives that are in line with your aims and values. We will also go through the need of evaluating and altering your objectives on a regular basis to reflect your changing requirements and circumstances.

7.4 Developing Self-Compassion:

Living with diabetes may be difficult at times, and self-compassion is crucial. We'll look at the notion of self-compassion and talk about ways to practice kindness, acceptance, and self-care. You may endure setbacks with resilience and keep a healthy connection with your diabetes management if you treat yourself with kindness and empathy.

7.5 Accepting Help and Community:

Long-term success requires maintaining a supporting network and interacting with the diabetic community. We'll talk about the relationships you've made, the assistance you've gotten, and how you may give back to those experiencing similar issues. You may gain strength, inspiration, and knowledge from the collective experiences of others by accepting assistance and actively engaging in the diabetic community.

7.6 Keeping Healthy Habits:

Maintaining the good behaviors you've formed along the way is critical to long-term blood sugar management. We will go through tactics for eating a healthy diet, getting enough exercise, dealing with stress, and sticking to drug regimes. Making these practices a part of your daily routine can guarantee your sustained success in regulating your blood sugar levels and general well-being.

Conclusion:

Chapter 7 represents the conclusion of your journey to living a balanced and meaningful life with diabetes. You have gained the skills and mentality required to handle the difficulties of blood sugar control with resilience and determination via introspection, gratitude, mindfulness, goal setting, self-compassion, and continual support. Remember that this is a lifetime commitment to your health and well-being, not a destination. Accept the lessons you've learned, appreciate your triumphs, and look forward with confidence and hope. You can live a lively, meaningful life with diabetes, and I wish you continued success on this transformational journey.

Looking Forward: Empowering Future Possibilities

Introduction:

In Chapter 8, we'll look forward and consider future options for regulating blood sugar levels and enjoying a satisfying life with diabetes. You have absorbed useful information, learned crucial skills, and formed a resilient and self-care mentality throughout this book. Now is the moment to look forward with hope, to arm yourself with the opportunities that lie ahead, and to begin on a road of sustained progress and well-being.

8.1 Embracing Diabetes Management Advances:

Diabetes care is a continually expanding subject, with new technology, drugs, and treatment techniques being created all the time. We will talk about how important it is to remain up to date on the newest advances in blood sugar management and to embrace new opportunities. You may benefit from the most recent technologies and tactics available by keeping open to new ideas and working closely with your healthcare team.

8.2 Leveraging Technology's Potential:

Technology is important in diabetes treatment because it provides creative ways to help with blood sugar control. We will look at how digital health tools, smartphone apps, and wearable devices may be used to check blood sugar, manage lifestyle behaviors, and access educational materials. Understanding how to use technology to your advantage might help you make more educated choices and remain on track with your diabetes care.

8.3 Education and Advocacy:

Educating and advocating for yourself and others is a powerful strategy to affect the future of diabetes treatment. We will talk about how important it is to raise awareness, advocate for better access to healthcare services, and participate in diabetes-related projects and research. You may have a positive influence on the diabetic community and help to advance the area of diabetes management by sharing your expertise and experiences.

8.4 Personal Development and Reinvention:

Diabetes provides opportunity for personal development and reinvention. We will look at how to embrace change, create new objectives, and uncover new hobbies and interests. You may tap into your inner strengths and embrace the opportunities for a full life outside the limits of diabetes by seeing it as a catalyst for personal growth.

8.5 Developing Resilience:

Resilience is a basic characteristic that enables people to overcome obstacles and flourish in the face of adversity. We will reflect on your resilience during this trip and provide methods for increasing this vital trait. You can negotiate the ups and downs of blood sugar control with confidence, flexibility, and a firm trust in your capacity to overcome hurdles if you cultivate resilience.

8.6 Rejoicing in Your Journey:

Chapter 8 finishes with a toast to your accomplishments so far. We will reflect on the progress you have made, the lessons you have learned, and the accomplishments you have reached. By recognizing and celebrating your progress, you may boost your motivation, strengthen your dedication to blood sugar management, and lay the groundwork for a future filled with health, pleasure, and contentment.

Conclusion:

In Chapter 8, we looked at the notion of anticipating and enabling future possibilities for regulating blood sugar levels and having a satisfying life with diabetes. You may begin on a path of sustained empowerment and well-being by embracing improvements in diabetes management, utilizing the power of technology, pushing for change, fostering personal development, and building resilience. Remember that you have the ability to influence your future and live a life that is full of pleasure, purpose, and optimum blood sugar management. As you go, embrace the chances that await you, and may your path be filled with limitless possibilities and a profound feeling of satisfaction.

Conclusion:

You have received a wealth of information and practical ways to empower yourself and live a healthy, meaningful life as a result of your quest to regulate your blood sugar level. We looked at the foundations of blood sugar control, the role of physical activity, stress management techniques, medication management, the importance of support systems and self-care, reflections on your journey, and looking ahead to future possibilities throughout this book.

You have learnt to make educated food choices that encourage stability and good health by understanding the influence of diet on blood sugar levels. Regular physical exercise has not only helped you regulate your blood sugar but has also enhanced your entire well-being. You have navigated the obstacles of diabetes with perseverance and a good mentality thanks to effective stress management practices.

You now understand the many drug alternatives accessible and the significance of following recommended regimens. The importance of support networks and self-care techniques in your diabetes journey has been highlighted, enabling you to establish a strong network and prioritize your mental and physical well-being.

Reflecting on your trip has given you the chance to appreciate your accomplishments and recognise your personal progress. Looking forward, you have the knowledge and skills to embrace diabetes management innovations, leverage the power of technology, and contribute to the diabetic community via advocacy and education.

Remember that regulating your blood sugar level is a lifetime responsibility as you finish this book. It requires continuous self-awareness, education, and modification. You will be well-prepared to manage the problems that may occur and grab the possibilities for a balanced and satisfying life if you use the methods and insights obtained throughout these chapters.

Always work closely with your healthcare team, test your blood sugar levels on a regular basis, and seek support from loved ones and the diabetic community. Your path is unique, and you can overcome challenges, attain optimum blood sugar management, and enjoy a life of health, happiness, and satisfaction with the information and empowerment you've learned.

Congratulations on your determination to regulate your blood sugar levels and live a healthy lifestyle. As you continue on your journey to long-term well-being, may this book serve as a guide and source of inspiration for you. I wish you a healthy, happy life with good blood sugar management.

www.ingramcontent.com/pod-product-compliance
Lightning Source LLC
Chambersburg PA
CBHW081854250726
48659CB00008B/2743